I Still Love You
The love story of an Alzheimer's caregiver

By

Jean Darby

ISBN: 0-75962-019-9

This book is printed on acid free paper.

1stBooks - rev. 10/2/01

I Still Love You is a tribute to Raymond Vern Darby Jr. who suffered from Alzheimer's and died on April 15, 1999.

It is an inspiring story of faith and courage that grew from notes kept by his wife. It is her hope that sharing their experience will bring comfort to others who cope with the mysterious disease.

Raymond was filled with life and spirit, walking four miles instead of one. He played tennis into his later years. Best of all, he loved to fly.

A fighter pilot of the best sort, he survived 100 missions over the Himalayas into China. A tiger of the 14th Air Force--that was Ray.

Ray...

    This is my way of telling you what happened.

It has been two months since you said good-bye. Or is it two years? Three? Maybe a dozen? My heart aches and time means nothing. I reach for you and my arms come back empty. I drift in space. There is no one to hold me now.

You had been ill for a long time when the doctor told me something was taking you. "It's a mystery," he said, "I don't know what it is."

I thought, it's angels, but I didn't tell him.

I kissed your forehead. You didn't stir, but I think you knew I was there. I believe you heard me say, "I love you."

They said you didn't understand, but I think you did. I couldn't have stood it if I hadn't believed God was keeping his promise. You were so peaceful, it seemed you were already beginning to heal.

I listened to your breathing slow--and slow. I hoped you knew how much I loved you.

I dared to wonder--could you recall the night we rode across the desert and promised to love forever? Could you remember how we held each other...the first time we made love--our first quarrel and how we made up?

Could you recall telling me our baby girl came from heaven?

That's what you said, and I cried.

Some people believed I took care of you for too long. They said I was brave, but they didn't know us. Dearly beloved, it was my privilege.

I miss you but I try not to cry. Crying would be unfaithful to what you believed.

You are with our Father in heaven. Your guardian angel hovers close by. And so I wait. And wait for that precious day when we meet again.

I had gone on an errand. You were alone. When I returned your face was pale. You seemed unsure, as if something had frightened you. You said, "I was talking on the telephone. Suddenly I couldn't speak. I couldn't write."

Had I known what lay ahead, my heart would have stopped.

#

A trip to the emergency room infuriated me. How could even a blustering doctor be so cruel? Without flinching he said, "It's the beginning of Alzheimer's."

I steeled. It couldn't be. It couldn't happen to someone so strong--so full of life--so mentally young.

We went home silently denying it all. The doctor had no proof. I knew it. He was wrong.

During the months that followed, you were weak. You slept a lot. You had trouble remembering, and you had trouble speaking. Words that you once knew were mysteriously gone. I began filling them in for you. I'd laugh and explain, "We're getting good at charades."

I told myself you'd had a slight stroke. We talked about it. "Of course, it was a stroke. You'd heal."

We continued our daily routine of meeting friends for lunch. Going to restaurants for our evening meal and attending small dinner parties. Life had changed only slightly even though you were unusually tired, even though you had trouble speaking.

You had another stroke. And another. You knew fewer words. Your memory grew worse. You couldn't remember what we had done, where we had gone or where you put your belongings. It was then I began to know how strong we had to be.

Medication was prescribed for Alzheimer's. I swore I would never tell you the name of your illness. That was a must. I would never tell.

Each night we held each other and said the Lord's prayer. That simple practice was part of the glue that had held us together for more than fifty years. We would begin. You'd forget. We'd laugh and start again. We'd kiss and say, "Goodnight." Sometimes I'd whisper, "I love you." You'd say, "That's good."

I knew you cared. *Oh how you cared!*

In the beginning I'd leave you for an hour or two. It was lunch with a friend, or an afternoon of bridge. I'd hurry home wondering how you were.

Had you needed me? How lonely had you felt? My heart pounded the message, *You mustn't be depressed.* Finally worry overtook the joy of going.

I'd stay home. I had to be with you.

5

#

There were days you went to a clinic for therapy. You would draw letters, and numbers. A young woman helped you with your speech and you were grateful for her patience. On the way home you'd buy a hamburger. It was *the* event of the day. For one brief hour you felt free. You drove yourself. You were independent.

Independent? *Oh my dear!* You who had managed the finances of the county's schools. You who had established an environmental camp for children, brought Head Start to the county and founded a school for pregnant girls. And you who spoke with eloquence to an auditorium filled with parents.

"Ladies and gentlemen," you said. "I give you the cutest kids in Shasta County." It was a Christmas program. I was so proud.

#

Home from therapy, I knew you were safe. I arranged your hamburger and fries on a T.V. tray, turned on a western movie and together we settled in for a quiet afternoon.

You would doze. Waken and look at me. Knowing I was there seemed incredibly important. Seeing me, you'd smile and go back to sleep. I stayed knowing you would wake again. I had to be there.

I could have read but something within kept me from the books I loved. You could no longer decipher words. You had been brutally robbed. How could I enjoy a book in front of you?

#

We went to the grocery store every day. You'd choose cinnamon graham crackers and vanilla ice cream. I'd ask what else you wanted. It was difficult for you to decide...a growing problem. Walking up and down the aisles we'd smile at each other as if to say *it's okay. We're together.* To myself I'd think, *we're making it.*

Some moments were more difficult than others.

Chills crawled up my spine when I'd hear, "Well hi there, Ray. I haven't seen you for a long time. How've you been?"

You'd stare unable to find the words you knew you wanted. Once familiar they were now lodged in, or shoved out of your brain. No matter how often it happened, the unexpected greeting remained a catastrophic hurt.

When I saw an acquaintance in the distance, I'd say, "Let's go. It's almost time for Mash," or, "The movie starts in fifteen minutes." I would hurry you out of the store and we'd head for the safety of our home.

#

Time passed.

All that you suffered grew worse, but there were windows that opened letting in bits of light. I wished some of them had remained closed.

One morning as I stirred hot cereal I heard you say, "I have Alzheimer's." Startled, I asked, "What makes you think that?"

"It says so here."

"I turned to see you holding your medication. "Here," you said. You showed me the bottle. "I have Alzheimer's, but not as bad as Polly."

#

I had entered a time of life I hadn't expected to experience. The hours were filled with emotions...despair, then victory, then something in between. My burden grew heavier. Again and again I asked myself if I would be strong enough.

Then quietly, as if on slippered feet, something wonderful began to happen.

Walking through our daily routine I experienced a new presence. It was as if I stepped into a place where I had never been. Suddenly it seemed I was surrounded by something soft. "Don't try to understand," whispered through my inner being. Suddenly, miraculously, I loved you more. I asked myself *how can it be?*

The days rolled one into another. Weeks stacked. Months collected and became years. You began to press your hand against your chest. Or was it your stomach? Your rib cage?

Did you feel pain? A dull hurt? An ache? You couldn't tell me how it felt, nor could you find its exact location. It came and went along with being cold, then hot. You put wraps on then immediately took them off. You looked perplexed. You also were in a world you had never before experienced. You didn't understand yourself. I struggled but did not know how to fix all that was going wrong. Only one thing was plain. You were getting worse. You were more confused. More dull. I reached harder to find the person you once were.

Again and again I hunted for your glasses, your hat, your coat. Again and again I'd repeated sentences you didn't understand. I told you again and again information you didn't remember. You'd say, "I don't know what I'd do without you." I'd shrug and say. "No problem," as my surprised mind focused on your sudden ability to speak.

It was my fault that we stopped seeing friends. I'd tell them, "Ray isn't able to go." I wondered if I was isolating us too soon. Was I being selfish? How many years would we be left to our own devices? I'd try to explain. "Ray is not able to visit. He doesn't understand. He can't respond."

I dared to ask, was I protecting you or me? Or was it something I did for us?

Secretly I admitted pride was mixed with sorrow. I had been married to a successful man. A prominent citizen, aggressive and creative. Suddenly you, my husband, my other half, was incapable of making the most simple decision...incapable of carrying on the most mundane conversation. You didn't care what you wore, or if your hair was combed. I felt unsure. Not proud.

Emotionally I choked. An inner voice screamed, *love...don't leave me now!*

Hurts came one after the other taking on their own personality, each more heart-wrenching than the one before.

#

Sitting beside you as you drove I realized we were traveling in an unsafe car. It came as a sudden revelation. *He's incompetent. Not fit.* Fatigue washed over me like a giant wave. My stomach grabbed. How could I say it? How could I who love you wield such a catastrophic blow? How could I deprive you of your last independence?

Frightening questions blasted my brain. *How much responsibility do I have to take? How much can I stand?* Then came the worst of all thoughts. *Am I reaching the limit of my strength? Am I caving in? Is my steel wall cracking?*

After days of emotional writhing, I weighed my strength against my love for you. I told myself one could not be stronger than the other. As long as love remained, I would protect you. Then I heard my mother's voice, "God will not ask you to do more than you are able."

I planted this thought in every crevice of my being and I asked myself again and again, *how can I keep you from hurting yourself, or someone else?*

The answer came in the middle of the night. It was clear and it seemed amazingly simple. I would tell our doctor of my concern. He would help. I was sure of it.

#

"Of course," he said. "That time has probably come. I'll have my nurse test him."

You failed. The doctor's words were blunt. Too quick. They almost stood alone repeating themselves in our hearts. "I'm notifying the DMV. You're not to drive."

If my heart could shout it would have screamed, f*orgive me dearly beloved. Please forgive me!*

You were shattered. Your feelings were so intense, we had to change physicians.

The DMV wrote a threatening letter demanding the return of your driver's license. Every part of my being grew angry as I wondered why you couldn't carry the small piece of paper in your wallet. The card was small and rumpled. What it stood for was gigantic. Even in your confused mind you knew you were forfeiting your identity. It was another way of saying I am no longer me.

I handed you your wallet and watched your pain, wishing I could change the inevitable.

After a long pause you slipped the little card out of its case. Your fingers moved slowly over the numbers and across your picture. You took one last look, then handed it to me.

#

I cried inside as I drove you to therapy. Your last vintage of freedom gone, I sensed hope disappearing.

Going to see the young woman who had helped you was no longer a joyful experience. Before many days passed, you quit.

Months later, during a quiet moment, I thought I heard you speak. I listened carefully to hear, "Remember how I drove to the hospital?"

My eyes filled with tears. A lump ached in my throat. I nodded thinking how strange that you suddenly recalled events, and even more strange that you found the right words.

Your return to near normalcy was rare. In spite of the little windows that opened, each day it became more apparent you were on a slippery slope heading for disaster. My heart cried, *our world is falling apart!*

#

We were more alone. One day you mumbled, "Remember when the tennis players asked me to breakfast?"

"I remember."

17

"Then they all did something else."

"I remember that, too."

"Nobody came."

Frantically I wondered what I could do to fill the holes that kept appearing in our lives. I thought, *if only the gaps were empty.* They were not empty. They were filled with torment.

My heart told me you needed more than me. You needed something else you could love. Something that would love you back. It would be there...always there for you.

I thought of your love for children. I remembered how you cared for little animals. That's it! A smile came sneaking as my mind raced. I'd get an animal. Something furry you could love. Something that wouldn't care if you didn't remember. *A puppy! That's it!* A little dog wouldn't notice how you tried to speak, but couldn't.

We drove to Sacramento and gave a young Chinese woman four hundred dollars. In return she let us take home a black Miniature Schnauzer. It was love at first sight. We called her Missy.

You gave Missy the best you had. Bites from your plate and walks down the road. In return she became your best friend cuddling beside you and letting you know that, to her, nothing was wrong. You were okay. Special.

#

The little dog helped, but it remained apparent that the slope was tilting. It was steeper. The downward slide brought constant surprises that jarred my confidence and made me wonder how well I was taking care of you.

One of those times happened when you looked away from our movie and said, "I need money."

For me it was like rolling a boulder into a cluster of pebbles.

I knew too well how you had managed our money. And, my darling, you did it so well. How could I tell you? How could I say *you don't know the difference in numbers? You don't know a ten dollar bill from a twenty, or a nickel from a dime?*

You held your wallet open and stared at its empty space, then at me.

My heart thumping, I wondered what you wanted to purchase. It crossed my mind that you might want to go somewhere. The thought of you wandering away frightened me. "Of course," I said and I gave you a five dollar bill and four ones.

#

During the evening we watched television in the family room. When you fell asleep, I'd go to our bedroom to prepare for the night. Exhausted I lay in bed, dozed and wakened often stepping to the door. I'd look down the hall and through the living room where I could see you sleeping. When the hours sneaked toward midnight I'd wake you.

Touching your knee, I'd say. "It's late. It's time to go to bed."

You would stir. Smile and follow me.

It was probably a foolish routine, but nothing about our lives was normal. What difference did it make?

But all was not well.

The night came when I wakened to hear pounding on the bedroom window.

My feet hit the floor and I ran to the family room. You weren't in your chair. You weren't in the bathroom. Not in the kitchen. My heart pounded. *What could have happened? Where could you be?*

21

I opened the door to the front yard and called into the night, "Where are you?"

Out of the darkness, you came. Frightened. Bewildered. "I got lost. I couldn't get home."

You'd been in front of our house--a house you'd lived in for more than forty years. You didn't recognize the light, the steps, the porch. You rang a neighbor's doorbell. You banged on her door. She had guided you down the steps and into the yard.

I helped you into bed with Missy cuddling close. I was embarrassed that you had frightened our neighbor and angry with myself. I should have known better. You must have wakened confused and gone out the back door. You could have wandered over the hill and fallen off a cliff. You could have been hurt on the highway. I had to watch more closely. My time alone had come to an end.

#

It was then that our daughter suggested we sell our home and move closer to her. "As a family we can work together," she said. "I can help you and I can help daddy."

I understood her concern but the thought of leaving our home seemed preposterous. We had lived on Pearl Street most of our married life. Our home had been purchased with a G I loan, easily paid for in our middle years. We'd added rooms. Decorated and redecorated.

We built a patio and had barbeques with special friends. We cheered the town's fireworks. It was where, on soft summer nights, I sat with you watching the stars and exchanging secrets that we held in our hearts.

Twenty-four hundred feet of memories stood on a hill over looking the town and the Sacramento river.

Now, our daughter was asking us to turn our backs on all we had known and reconstruct our lives in another town. It seemed incredibly reckless.

But time has a way of changing things.

As you became increasingly dependent, as we were more isolated, the thought of moving surfaced oftener.

How could I tell you what I was thinking?

Day after day I grappled with the mystery of your mind. Again and again I asked myself if you would understand. Would you realize we were selling our home? Actually leaving? Going away? That we could no longer sit together in the family room eating hamburgers? That we would not watch television in our familiar place, or go to bed

in the room you loved? Would it be a surprise
when a big truck backed down the driveway?
When strangers picked up our furniture and carried
it out of the house? How would you react when
books you treasured disappeared into boxes?
Would all of these make you more confused and
more unhappy?

How could I risk another unknown? Another
place where we had never been? Deep inside, I
feared the frightening anger which so often
accompanies Alzheimer's. Did I have the courage
I would need? How much was I willing to
gamble?

#

My daughter and her family moved into a new
home on four acres. Next door three acres stood
waiting for us.

25

Beau (our college-age grandson) was adamant. "The property will be gone. If you want it, buy it now."

Beyond worrying about the drastic change in our lives was the overwhelming realization that I had only recently been in charge of the checkbook that paid the family bills. I struggled with insurances and taxes and when the car had to be lubed. There were those occasions when I lifted the bills from the mailbox, my stomach turned over. Had I forgotten something? Did I have enough money? The frightening thought of making a mistake was a hound at my heels.

So how could I who had somehow survived living in an emotional drought of finances sell a house, purchase property and undertake building a new home? All of this while taking care of a husband who might not understand any of it. Piled on these thoughts was the realization that I was dealing with an ailment that no lay person, no physician, no psychiatrist completely understood. There was no number I could call. No one to tell me: *do this and this will happen.* I worried that when the moving process began you might suddenly realize what was happening. You might become frightened and rebel. What would I do then?

#

I looked at you and wondered if you could recall the day we first discussed moving?

We sat together in the family room with Missy sleeping in your lap. I told you, "Diane would like us to be near her. She believes we should live next door. We could go to Buck's football games. It would be nice to watch Britt play soccer."

You nodded.

I wondered how much you understood.

"Would you like to take a ride? We could see the kids and look at the property."

You said, "If you want to," and picked up Missy. Of course she'd come with us.

#

We walked over the land and I watched you closely. Something about you made me think you would accept the idea of being here. I edged closer to making a decision, but, like a giant raven, the unknown hovered. How much did you understand?

There were other problems that concerned me.

Pulling up roots. Creating a new lifestyle along with learning about loans, interest rates and working with contractors demanded qualities I was

not sure I had. I would need supernatural strength.
Would it be there for me?

#

We were close in bed. A ribbon of light lay
across your face. So familiar. So much that I had
loved. Into the night I whispered, "Can you trust
me enough?" It was all right that you didn't
answer because I knew the reason for your silence.

After a long while I whispered our prayer then,
feeling a bit of satisfaction, fell asleep.

#

I must have made the decision during my
unconscious hours. When I wakened I was in a
planning mode. I knew what I had to do.

Events moved quickly.

I hired someone to paint the carport and the side of the house where the summer sun had done the most damage. Plants that grew down the hill were trimmed, closets rearranged, windows cleaned and carpets shampooed.

I purchased the land in Red Bluff then telephoned a realtor who put our house on the market. Three days later the home we had laughed and loved in, where we had joyfully brought up our daughter, belonged to a stranger. I hoped the quick sale was a signal that my inner compass was leading me in the right direction.

In spite of my gaining confidence, one haunting question remained. Did you have any idea of events that would follow?

Critical decisions had to be made so I fought to keep at bay the sinking feeling that threatened to steal my courage. I had to move on. The clock was ticking.

#

I could no longer question my decision. I had jumped into a stream that raced toward a cliff. I had to find a place for us to live.

For Rent signs were prevalent, but I quickly learned that apartment hunting with a Schnauzer does not limit one's choices, it eradicates them. Weighing my options, I made an unexpected choice.

It was a blustery afternoon. While you and Missy slept, I hurried to Cousin Gary's RV lot.

I explained our situation to a sales person who seemed comfortable with himself and with his work. "I'm looking for a trailer that my husband and I can live in?"

"You're going to live in it permanently?"

"For five months."

When he seemed confused I said, "While we build a house. We're moving."

He was certain he had the perfect vehicle for us.

It was 29 feet long. Not class "A" but we could make it work.

Feeling suddenly up and in control I said, "I'll take it." I wrote a check for ten thousand dollars and he promised to place our new home on a cement slab behind our daughter's house.

Pulling onto the highway, I felt heady. *Step one. Mark it off. I did what I had to do. It has to be right.*

But how would I tell you? Where were you in your thinking? How fuzzy was what you thought? How plain? One question hammered through me. *Where are you?* It was a constant beat. A bongo drum I couldn't stop hearing.

I lived with the fear of stumbling or making a catastrophic mistake that I...we could not recover from.

#

I pulled into the carport, stopped the car and sat quietly gathering my courage. Finally I looked toward the house. "Get out of the car," I said. "Face whatever you have to face. " I opened the back door. You looked at me and Missy sat up.

My mind turned a corner and I quickly asked, "Are you okay?" I don't know why I said it but I found myself asking again and again if you were all right. It seemed you were changing. Looking more worried. Perhaps in some misguided way I thought I could help.

In the beginning, you would say, "I guess." Later it was, "Not really."

But there it was. Another change. No matter how I tried to deny it, you were different. Something else was bothering you. A different place was hurting. You couldn't tell me how or where. *So why did I ask?*

"I have something to tell you."

A slight smile.

"I bought a trailer. We'll put it in Diane's backyard. We'll live in it while our house is being built."

Your smile was more definite. I was off the hook. I breathed easier thinking it was another positive sign.

Suddenly I was overwhelmed with respect for you. Through the haze I saw your dignity. Your self control. I felt you knew I was doing the best I could. Quickly I was on the floor in front of you.

"We'll have a good time," I said. "Really, we will." I took your hand as I tried not to cry.

"Honey, I love you. I appreciate your helping me."

I wondered if you understood.

#

You were concerned about our possessions. I tried to assure you. "We'll take them with us. I promise."

"Even that?" You pointed to a chair.

"Yes. Even that."

"Even that?" You pointed to a table.

"Even that."

#

My work was cut out for me and I had to move quickly sorting belongings that we had collected for forty years.

Cupboards were jammed memories: motorcycle helmets, skis and rubber rafts once used at the lake. There were picnic baskets, and small-sized boots which no longer fit my college-age grandsons. There were boxes filled with a conglomeration of articles I mentally labeled junk. It became obvious that over a span of four decades the years were recorded in boxes and on shelves. My task was to get all the unneeded items out of the house. I had to do this without frightening you.

I collected outdated books on education and health and novels we wouldn't read again. While you slept, I carried them around the outside of the house and stacked them in the trunk of the car. Later they were delivered to the library or secondhand stores.

I filled garbage bags with items that had no value. In the late hours of night I dragged them down the stairs and threw them into the trash.

Little by little most of what we didn't want or need was eliminated.

You never noticed that so many things were taken away. I was grateful. You had to believe I was keeping my promise. Your possessions were going with us.

#

Finally the momentous day came. We were leaving our home. I heard the truck shifting as it turned the corner. I listened as it rumbled toward our house. *Stay strong!* I begged it of me and I begged it of you. *Stay strong! Please! Please stay strong!*

The truck loomed large and turned around in the culdesac. Missy barked and ran to the door. I hurried to where you were sitting in the family room and sat next to you. "Honey."

You looked bewildered.

I touched your knee. "The truck is here. Men are coming into the house. They are going to put our furniture on the truck."

"Now?"

"Right now?" You looked frightened.

"They'll keep it while we build our new home. When our house is finished, they will bring it to us."

"You're sure?"

"I'm sure."

We stood and walked toward the door. I opened it and five young men stepped into the living room. I told you, "It's okay. They'll take good care of everything."

You watched quietly while the men wrapped our belongings and sealed up boxes. You stood in the front yard and watched tables, chairs and our bedroom set disappear under brown blankets. You saw when they were shoved into the truck. Fears of your rebellion had been in vain.

When the house was empty and the movers were gone, we walked from room to room saying good-by to a lifetime of memories. Memories that belonged only to us. I kissed your cheek and thought *thank you.* "Let's go," I said. "Diane is waiting."

#

I feared this might be a day of panic. A day when my heart would race and I'd blink back tears. The same haunting question was with me again stalking my every move. *What goes on in your brain?*

I clenched the steering wheel and turned to see you smiling. In that split second I knew you trusted me. Around a knot in my throat I said,

"It's going to be all right. We're going to have a good time."

"We'll see Diane?"

"She'll be waiting."

You looked at me and smiled again, a spark dug up from the past. Haltingly you asked, "You bought a trailer?"

"That's right."

"Just went out and bought it?"

"Yes."

"You wrote a check?"

I knew you saw the difference in what I had done. Me making the decision. Me writing a check for ten thousand dollars...coming home and announcing the purchase. A slit of a window had opened in your brain and let you know what was happening.

I said, "I love you" and the lump grew bigger. I hurried to talk.

"We should get to Diane's before the trailer arrives."

You were silent. I wondered *has the window closed? That small bit of light disappeared so soon?*

I told myself not to fuss. It had been a blessing.

When we pulled into our daughter's driveway, the truck and trailer were close behind.

"There it is. Our new home."

Everyone was there. Our grandsons: Brooks, Beau, Buck, Britt and their parents Bob and Diane. It was a day of celebration. We had a plan. We were making it work.

I stood by you as the truck maneuvered the trailer onto the slab.

"That's it. Our new home."

We were excited.

Electricity and water were hooked up. Moving quickly we unloaded the car. Dishes, pots and pans, towels, blankets, and pillows, were stashed in tiny cupboards. We put together wardrobe closets and stood them in the garage. An hour later our clothes were organized and hung.

I was proud of our efficiency and proud of you. You were with me, not rebelling. Not acting out fear. I felt the discipline you practiced for a lifetime was with you now. Disabled you were somehow still in control. I asked myself, *Is that possible? Could someone with Alzheimer's do that? Practice self control?*

No one may ever know. But with every heart beat I said, "Thank you."

Helping each other, we were on our way to a new life. We were together.

#

The family rallied around. Their excitement underscored the positive aspects of our journey.

"Come with me." It was our son-in-law speaking. "I'll show you the boundaries of your land."

We trudged over three acres of grass and star thistle with Missy close behind. We speculated on where we would place our new home. I knew that you understood what we were doing. You wanted to know something about the house and once again I showed you its picture.

I'd found it in a magazine. Two story. Thirty-three hundred square feet. Why so big?

I never told you, but we, all of us in the family wanted to keep you home. No matter how ill you became, somehow, someway, we would keep you with us. It was our goal. Our heartfelt determination. No one could take care of you as we could. No one could love you as we did. Therefore, I chose a house with a downstairs master bedroom. We needed an upstairs that I could move into if you required more help at night.

We gave the house plans to Sequoia Builders. Dave Gilmore would place our new home next door to our daughter's. It was a natural choice since he had been Diane's contractor.

You sat with us as we discussed the floor plan, fixtures and the direction of the house, but you did not participate. It could have been a lonely trip had I not felt your patience, and perhaps a small amount of admiration. One thing was certain. You loved me for what I was trying to do.

Sometimes I turned to you almost forgetting that we could not share on a grown-up level. I could not tell you what the house would cost. I could not tell you how I handled the money paying cash for certain items to keep the price of the house down. It never failed to seem unreal, that you were unconcerned with the money we received for our home and the cost of rebuilding. Apparently you had no fear of debts or overspending. All that worry was gone.

We shared little things. The color of the house, which room was for your airplane pictures and TV. Which was my study. You only listened as I told you. Where things were, or what I planned made no difference.

Sometimes I wondered why I didn't feel more lonely. I asked myself *why am I not crying? Why am I not exhausted...asking for a drug to calm my nerves?* Secretly I knew. A quiet place was deep within me. Holding steady.

One day rolled into another and as each task presented itself, I solved it the best I could.

#

We had breakfast in the trailer. Took rides and ate lunch in a variety of restaurants. You could not read the menu but you looked at the pictures and I made suggestions. As time went on it became more difficult for you to eat. I was careful with what we ordered and I helped you more.

Diane cooked dinner for everyone. In the beginning we dined with her family, but soon carried our meals to the trailer where we watched television. It was a cozy time. Just the two of us eating on T V trays, sharing a movie and bites with Missy.

Sometimes I wondered if you could follow the story. I wondered how much you understood about the characters. I sensed a change as you struggled to ask me more of what happened. Who he was and where did she come from? Was this another way you were failing? The thought of you growing further away from me never failed to be frightening.

You couldn't converse. You couldn't read, write, or drive the car. Eating in restaurants became increasingly difficult and you could only walk short distances. If your ability to enjoy television should disappear what would we have left?

#

Missy slept with us in a double bed at the end of the trailer. The person who lay against the outside wall wrestled with being cold. The other person had to be crawled over. The arrangement was definitely inconvenient so you decided to sleep on the couch. This change worked well until the night something terrible happened in your brain.

Suddenly you were standing, shaking your head, making wild noises. You beat your fists against the walls, thrashed the blankets and dragged them down the hall. You banged against the stove and hit the refrigerator.

I screamed, "What are you doing?"

You ground your teeth and threw yourself against the cupboards.

"Please come back!"

You mumbled and kept walking.

Fright overcame me. I yelled again, "What are you doing?"

You whipped the blankets harder, tossed them on the table and crawled on top of them.

I screamed, "Don't! The table will break. Please! Please don't!"

You mumbled something like, "Sleeping here."

"The table won't hold you! It will break!"

You fell back. You had no pillow and your feet hung off the end.

"You can't sleep there!"

Your face contorted and your eyes filled with torment, you hit the wall and shot me a wild look.

Suddenly you seemed bigger and stronger. I didn't know you. Horror stories broke loose in my mind. *He didn't recognize his wife. He backed her against the wall. Hit her. Would you do that?* My heart pounded. I wasn't sure I could cope.

I hid my face in my hands, trying not to look, trying not to know what was real. When I dared to glance between my fingers, I shuddered. The terrifying look in your eyes was still there. I dropped my hands and wailed, "Honey. Please. Let me help you."

"You can't."

It was a knife in my heart.

49

"Nobody can help me."

It was another window. I didn't want to see in. "Let me try."

You stared as if struggling to think.

"Please come to bed."

Miraculously your torment began to fade. A tide going out, you softened. Together we gathered the blankets and put them on the couch. I covered you, kissed your forehead and brushed my hand across your cheek. When you closed your eyes I lay down on the bed frightened and exhausted. I stayed awake listening for your every move, at the same time wondering if this was the beginning of a new behavior.

Or was it something passing through? Another stroke, or some other traumatic change taking place in your brain?

I recalled a night in Redding when you shut the bathroom door and couldn't find your way out.

When I discovered you, you had taken all the towel racks off the walls.

Thinking about it now, I remember you were always taking things apart.

#

Were these happenings caused by a storm in your brain--a tornado come to destroy?

When the sun came up, your mad behavior was gone. I crawled across the bed and lifted the shade. "The contractor is on the lot. Let's help him decide where to put the house."

#

After much discussion and drawing lines in the dirt, the contractor and I agreed on the distance from the road, and the angle of our new home.

You remained placid. You had nothing to offer. You made no complaints.

"It's going to be beautiful," I said.

You nodded and I hoped you thought so too.

Every morning we checked to see if the workmen had arrived. I'd go to the window and call, "They're here," I'd tell you how many had come. Every day we walked together inspecting the job. We went from room to room our imaginations playing games as we placed furniture and pictured colors. I told you again and again which room was for your airplane pictures, that my study was next door. Again and again I told you which room was ours. We climbed the stairs to look out from the bedroom windows. I watched you closely fearing you might fall as, at first, there was no rail. Going down you'd sit, sliding from step to step. I'd watch, my heart aching, but still feeling pride. You were doing so well. Trying so hard.

"It's going to be beautiful." I repeated myself again and again.

#

Diane was wonderful. She helped as promised, going over bills, selecting wallpaper, carpet and tile. The very best in her came out to rescue me from moments when I became overwhelmed with contracts for cement and landscaping. How much did I need? What does one do with three acres? It was especially difficult for a person who had lived on a pie-shaped lot on the top of a hill.

Together we watched you grow worse. She'd say, "You're doing great, mother."

#

Winter winds shook the trailer. Rain pelted. You worried about the propane. We couldn't be cold. We were dependent on Diane's family to lift the tanks and help us keep them filled. The rugged weather forced us to make other arrangements about the sewer. Continually I was reminded that every decision fell on me. If mistakes were made, it was my fault. Because of all the work and inconvenience, I feared the day would come when you would say we should have stayed home. I dared not dwell on the thought.

And still you changed.

You were less steady on your feet, less capable of handling the trailer door. You were more apt to slip on the steps. It was another sign of your downward slide. *What could we do? How could we stop it?*

Diane took us to a doctor that was just right for you. He listened when you tried to speak. He was patient when you tried to tell him where you hurt. There was nothing anyone could do. The disease had been put in motion. It was driven by its own force.

#

Then, as if a miracle had happened, the house was up. Windows were in. Stucco was painted white proudly dotted with blue shutters and door. Tile shown in four bathrooms, the carpets were in. We had a home. Our furniture was coming. Our hearts were ablaze.

We waited for the big truck to fill the road in front of our house, then turn in. Finally, "Here it comes. It's here. The truck is here!"

I had planned where the furniture would fit. As quickly as each piece was brought into the house, it was put where it belonged. At the end of the day, we were in our new home. After forty some years our address had changed.

I looked about the rooms. Our familiar belongings brought warmth to my heart. I felt secure and strangely loved. We had made it. Together we did what we had to do. Together we had done that which seemed impossible.

You wanted to know where we would sleep.

Again I showed you.

"In our bed?"

"Together in our bed."

"But…"

"I'll put on the sheets and blankets. Our pillows are in the box. I'll get them out."

"We'll eat?"

"In here." We walked into the kitchen.

#

A couch and a love seat were angled together in the living room. During the day you'd lie on the couch. I'd be near you on the love seat. We watched westerns. Visited as much as we could. Wiled away the hours together. Always together. I wondered how much this had to do with your courage. Our smiling. Our touching.

As I remember it now, if I walked into another room, you were behind me. I'd hear you say, "There you are."

I had to be with you.

#

In the morning I'd prepare your shower and lay out your clothes.

You always wanted things that were the same. I knew they had to be comfortable. You were hurting more. Holding your chest. Making me wonder what was happening when tests proved there was no heart trouble. Nothing wrong with your lungs. What was it?

I'd select a pair of shoes, but instead of putting them on, you'd come to the living room walking slowly, stooped, worried and hugging an armload of misfits.

The muscles grabbed in my chest. *Not again!* I sat quietly holding my head. *Why does he do this? I laid out shoes that went together.*

You fumbled with oxfords, sandals, and boots as I gathered my strength, thinking *I have to be patient. He doesn't know what he's doing.* When my breathing became more even, I'd say, "Let me help you."

You were angry. Frustrated. "What's wrong?"

"They don't go together."

"What don't?"

"Let me show you."

You'd watch.

"These two match. You wore them yesterday. They were comfortable. You liked them."

You'd lean back and hold your head.

I changed your shoes.

The slope was getting steeper. You were slipping faster.

I felt incapable. I should have known better. All those shoes on the shelf were confusing. I should be able to anticipate these problems.

I was less amazed when you couldn't put on your shirt.

"Here's the sleeve. Can you put your arm in the sleeve?"

Your body was stiff. Your arm didn't twist the right way. You didn't know what to do. I didn't know how to help. Such a simple thing. How could it be? I wanted to throw myself on the bed and cry, but caving in was out of the question. I had to be strong.

I helped with your pants. They had to be loose. You were hurting.

Again and again I wondered why. More often I asked, "Are you okay?"

More often you said, "No."

You had trouble eating and I began to feed you. Your eyes were dull, but something about you was still there. A softness. A silent acknowledging that I was holding the spoon, offering you something you liked. In some small way we were still together living out our role as husband and wife. Mr. and Mrs. Raymond Darby entering our fifty-ninth year of marriage. It could not have been any other way.

We were back in the living room watching television. I wasn't sure if you remembered seeing the movie. You didn't say. I didn't ask.

Everything about you said, "I need you." Even in the silence I heard, "Don't leave me."

"I won't. I promise."

The day came when I was afraid to take you to the grocery store. You wouldn't stay in the car. You didn't want to come with me. Leaving you home was impossible.

I made quick trips picking up a few things, sometimes with you beside me. Sometimes while you waited in front of the store. The road I traveled was filled with signs that spelled DANGER AHEAD.

Frightening thoughts haunted me. *Soon will you not know who I am? How we loved? How we suffered?*

I'd waken frightened.

Is this the day? The worst day of my life ? The day I look into your eyes and realize I have become a stranger?

Along with these fears was the growing question *how could I keep our household going when I couldn't make a trip to the grocery store, the pharmacy, or bank?*

Your behavior became more complex. You would wear two hats. You told the mail person you'd bring her coffee. I was embarrassed. I hurt for you.

It was time to take the next step.

Jo to the rescue.

She was a wonderful woman who had experience taking care of elderly patients. She would shop, clean, cook and she helped to gird me against the frightening disease that stole my joy. Just seeing her enter the driveway lifted my load.

She came with a smile and often a bag full of furniture polish, laundry soap and groceries she knew we needed.

It was the beginning of March and we began taking notes on your behavior. It may seem cruel, but we did it only as a reminder. We needed facts to tell the doctor.

On March fifth Jo wrote:

Papa is confused. He keeps asking where the man went that was sitting on the couch.

He took the little table beside the couch and held it up in the air. He asked me what it was and he wanted to know where it went.

I put the table behind the couch and he went to the garage and tried to lift the door.

On March seventh I wrote:

Ray

Up at five. Crashed into the wall coming back from the bathroom.

Left water running on bathroom counter. Tried to clean it up. Everything wet.

Angry. Went back to bed.

Wanted to get in the shower with his clothes on.

When I asked him to join me by the fire, he yelled, "No!"

When I said, "Let me help you," he screamed, "You can't help me!"

It was midnight when you began walking. I pled with you, "Please. Come back to bed."

You kept walking. You slipped. You fell between the toilet and the wall. Around a lump in my throat I told you, "I can't pick you up."

After struggling with the bar and toilet seat, you managed to get on your feet. I begged you to come back to bed, but you kept walking. I felt my sphere of strength unwinding.

It wasn't that I didn't love you. You were right when you said, "You can't help." You had traveled beyond the intelligence God gave me. I was a small vessel bobbing on a stormy sea without compass or rudder.

But even though I felt the blackbirds hover, even though I heard the solemn drum--deep inside, holding fast, was the quiet place. A reservoir still and steady.

Your agonizing nights multiplied. You walked incessantly. You grabbed furniture. Pushed chairs. You urinated on the cupboards. *Oh my darling!* I couldn't protect you enough.

All day long I had to be where you could see me, and where I could see you. When you were alone, you had panic attacks.

Bob told me of a young man who would help us at night. He could be trusted and I could rest. It seemed impossible another problem was being solved. Greg came capable and smiling. We couldn't have made a better choice.

The doctor prescribed drugs to keep you calm. They didn't work. You grew more angry. More agitated. My heart cried, *where are we going? What turbulent ocean are we headed for?*

It was in the midst of this typhoon that I went to see a long time friend and business partner. During our conversation, suddenly as if propelled by some spiritual access, he asked, "Has Ray joined the Catholic church?"

I was stunned. *What made him ask?* He must have caught my surprise because he said, "Ray often told me he had wanted to join the church."

How could I have missed it?

We had begun our married life as Methodists. Later we became Congregationalists. And now this!

John was a devoted Catholic. As he spoke I recalled you telling me that you were envious of his faith. Since you were a bible reading Protestant who loved the Lord, I had not taken your comments seriously. I faintly recalled saying something that now seems flippant. "It's too late for us. There's too much to learn." How could I have been so blind, so short sighted?

John was speaking. "Ray always wanted to hear about..."

As he spoke, my mind raced--*the Catholic church. Ray wants to join the Catholic church.*

67

Diane, Bob and the boys are devoted to Catholicism. Why hadn't I realized?

That evening I told Diane what happened. Was it too late? We had to know. Diane contacted her priest and explained our situation. It was Father Michael who came to the house.

Suddenly you were more calm.

I leaned close to you, my eyes full of tears. "Father Michael has come to help us."

"Really?"

"I told him you wanted to join the Catholic church. He said you could."

Your eyes brightened. There was a smile on your lips. It was another window. Another streak of light. *He knows! He knows what's happening!*

You took communion. We held hands and tears rolled down my cheeks as we said, "Our Father Who Art In Heaven."

You wanted to know about me. Why hadn't I been included?

Father Michael's response was definite. "Easter Sunday. Your wife will join Easter Sunday."

He understands! It's a miracle!

So quickly you changed. Easter Sunday came and you couldn't be with me. I stood alone at the front of the sanctuary, a lump aching in my throat and my eyes blinking back tears. Oh how I wanted you beside me, holding my hand, sharing this miraculous moment.

#

Every day you were different from the one before. Now you would eat ice cream and share your spoon with Missy. A bite for you, then a bite for the Schnauzer. My first reaction was *no don't!*

But I managed to quietly observe you in your new world. You and your little dog were caring for each other in the manner both of you understood. What difference did it make of germs or disease? You already had the worst there was.

You hurt more and you were either hot or cold though the temperature in the house had not changed. You cringed at the thought of bed because the chilly sheets were uncomfortable. I began warming them with a hot pad.

I'd say, "It's better now. It will be all right."

You'd shake your head.

"Please. Feel it. See how warm it is."

I'd help you get ready for the night. Sometimes you'd agree to put on pajamas. Other times you'd change the top. There were times when you crawled into bed fully dressed.

I was afraid you'd be uncomfortable. The behavior seemed strange, but again I told myself, "This is what he wants. What does it matter?"

You grew increasingly stiff. You'd get on the bed as if to lie on your back then stop half way down, leaving your head in the air.

"Honey, please try. Try to put your head on the pillow."

You wouldn't move.

"Here," I said patting a specific spot. "It's soft. Put your head down here."

You didn't respond.

I'd try harder. "See this. It's your pillow. Put your head on the pillow."

I didn't know if you couldn't, or if you didn't understand. I didn't know how to help more, so I'd add another pillow folding them both, building them up to reach you. "Try to relax."

Then I'd think, *what made me give such foolish directions? Your body is stiff. Something terrible is happening to you.*

Your sleeping habits changed. You'd go to bed at eight o'clock, sleep until midnight then get out of bed. I'd open my eyes and see you, head down, fists closed, striding toward the door. My heart sank. *Not again! Not another horrible night!*

"Where are you going?"

What monstrous thing has got your mind?

You'd walk, and walk, and walk, and walk. You'd grab a chair and drive it around the room.

"Please don't!"

You kept on walking. Shoving. Pushing, grinding your teeth.

"Please! Come with me! Please get back in bed!"

It was a relentless force turned loose inside you. When I screamed, "Stop!" You said, "I can't," and I believed you.

You were a stranger disturbed beyond all reason. Jerking, walking, mumbling. Hour after hour I tried to reason with you and I tried to stop the destruction. It was no use. I should have known better.

You had left me. To you I was no longer your provider, your helpmate. You had departed from the sphere of our togetherness. You suffered from an insidious unknown that made you wild. I longed for daylight to turn my black windows gray. Instead the night seemed to go on forever. I praying for guidance and Missy hiding in her box.

"Please let me help you."

It was too late. The place you occupied was too complex. We had worked our way beyond our understanding.

I was frantic. *What do I do now?*

Shaking inside, I struggled to remain calm. There had to be an answer.

I had to find a way to take care of you.

Strangely, when I needed for you to sleep more, you slept less. You walked inside the house, then outside tramping three acres, plowing through dirt and weeds with me close behind making sure you didn't wander away.

Again and again I asked, "Please come with me. Come in the house."

You said, "I can't."

I believed you.

You were a stranger disturbed beyond all reason, jerking, walking, mumbling.

I had to have some relief so Jo agreed to spend longer hours with us.

I had hoped that would free me to go to the grocery store and take a walk with Missy, but you refused to stay alone with Jo. When I left the house, you went next door to be with Diane.

But Jo was needed. Having her in the house not only kept us clean and organized, I turned to her for added strength.

When Greg arrived at midnight, I went upstairs to sleep.

I chose midnight because that was when you usually wakened. Then came the night when you broke the rule.

It was eleven o'clock when you kicked back the covers and hit the floor walking. I rolled out, screaming, "Please don't. Please come back to bed."

You kept going.

I followed you into the living room.

You grabbed a chair and drove it back through the bedroom into the bathroom and straight for the shower door.

"Stop! Please stop! It will break! I took hold and pulled. It was a contest of wills and physical strength. I imagined you falling through the glass. I saw you bleeding. Then the chair turned and it was myself in danger. I glanced at the clock. Eleven twenty. *Greg come early! Please come early!*

We fought like two angry animals. Pulling. Tugging. Screaming at each other. It was a battle lost. You had crashed on the bottom of the slippery slope.

Finally I heard Greg open the front door. *Thank God! Thank God!*

"I'm so glad to see you! He's having a terrible night."

I went upstairs and crawled into bed too tired to cry and too exhausted to wonder about tomorrow.

#

When the sun came up, Greg and I had a cup of coffee. I dared to ask. "How was he?"

He smiled, "Okay."

"Did he go to bed?"

"He wouldn't stay."

"He walked?"

Greg nodded.

"All night?"

"I just got him down."

I hated to see Greg go. It would be four hours until Jo came.

You could no longer feed yourself and you refused foods. I'd offer you something you liked. You'd shake your head.

Diane said, "Daddy won't live long, he's beginning to shut down. It's a sign," she said, "he's getting ready to leave."

I didn't want to listen, but I did. Looking at our scoreboard of life, we were down to zero.

You had trouble getting to the bathroom on time. Making the problem worse, undressing and dressing were increasingly difficult. You could not follow the simplest instruction like, lift your foot. Your body continued to stiffen. The more confused you became, the more trouble I had helping you.

You continued to hurt more and still you couldn't tell me where. I looked for clothes that would not fit tight against your body. I thought I had found the answer when I brought home soft jersey pants with a drawstring. But you were irritated by the rope-like pieces that hung from your waist. You insisted that I take them off.

It was then, as we lay on our touching couches, I heard you say, "I'd like to stand up right here, right now and die."

Through the rubble in your brain did another streak of light come, a glimpse of reality? Did you suddenly realize the bare undeniable truth of how far you had fallen? And you spoke! How did you find the words? Where had they been hiding?

I closed my eyes and wished I could shut off my brain. After a time of weighty silence, I heard myself say, "I know."

We lay quietly searching our thoughts. *How clear were yours in that flash of light? And now are they gone? Have they disappeared into that abyss I can not reach? Dearly beloved where are you?*

#

And still you changed.

I handed you your toothbrush. You brushed the air in front of your mouth. I hurt to see such a frightening difference.

My body chilled as I realized you didn't know where your teeth were.

Had you forgotten the word, or was there something missing in association?

Why did I ask? It didn't matter. You were lost. But you did remember me.

I was so grateful.

I turned on the water in the shower and put the soap in your hand. You washed the walls. I shouldn't have been surprised. But I was.

I helped the best I could, but I was awkward. Please know, please always remember that I loved you.

#

Our lives were out of control. I had to have more help.

Bob, Diane and I took you to the doctor's office. He said, "It's a matter of medication. We have to get his medication adjusted."

"How can we do that?"

"In the hospital. It should only take two or three days."

I was overjoyed. You would be more quiet. I would have a measure of peace. I didn't realize we were entering another new place--a slice of our lives where I didn't want to go.

The drive to the hospital was short, just across town. We drove into the parking lot and attendants met us with a wheelchair. You stood, then I realized you weren't going to sit. My heart pounded. *Why is he so stiff?*

A giant of a man took hold of you. He forced you to bend. I wanted to scream *stop!* He didn't stop. He pushed you into the chair.

You pressed your fist against your chest. I bit words I didn't want to think, "You're hurting him!" I wanted to rush to your side, but I couldn't. The big man took you down the hall, away from me.

I turned to Diane. "Did you see how stiff Daddy is?"

She nodded.

"What do you think is happening?"

"I don't know. Nobody knows."

We sat in a small, closed room. After a lengthy discussion with hospital administrators it was determined that you couldn't stay. It seemed you weren't their exact kind of patient. They couldn't help you. They didn't want to try. I could hardly bear listening to their cold words. I wondered how much you understood.

Our senses dragging we climbed in the car while Diane telephoned your doctor. She came back saying, "We're going to St Elizabeth's."

I told you, "Your doctor is at another hospital. He said he could help you."

You drew your fingers into fists. You ground your teeth. You pressed your arm against your body. I felt your pain--the dagger inside you.

"The doctor will help," I said again hoping that I told the truth. And hoping that you understood how much I wanted it to happen.

At this hospital you went through the same routine. You were pushed into a wheelchair and taken away. But your doctor said you could stay. Nurses aids speedily prepared your room.

We waited in the hall. When I saw you again, you looked pale against white sheets. Pale, but agitated. You clawed the air. You drew your legs back and forth on the sheet. Through tears I told you, "You'll feel better soon. The doctor will help." I kissed your forehead and whispered, "I love you." I told you, "You're here to get your medication adjusted. You'll be home in three days."

What did he hear? What does he know?

I pled with the doctor. "Please give him something to stop his hurting?" When he seemed puzzled, I said. "Look at him. He's jerking and pulling the covers. He can't lie still. Please give him something to settle him down."

"I will," he said, "I promise."

I leaned over you, crying. "I'll be back soon." I kissed you. It was hard to believe that you might not know I was there, trying desperately to help.

Bob went to his office. Diane and I went to a restaurant to sit quietly toying with food we didn't feel like eating.

Diane said, "Daddy won't live very long."

"It will be a blessing--but having him go seems so..."

"Unfair."

"He tried so hard to take care of himself."

"I know."

"Are you finished? Is that all you can eat?"

"I want to get back to the hospital."

We paid the bill and were on our way, silence hanging around us like a heavy shroud. We parked. Entered the hospital and began our long walk down the hall to your room. Getting there seemed an eternity.

When we stepped inside you were writhing on the bed, drawing your legs up, shoving them down. Your face contorted you jerked your head back and forth on the pillow. You reached for me and took hold of my hand, saying, "Honey, honey!"

I burst into tears and ran into the hall to the nurse's station. Pushing my way through a circle of visitors, I said, "The doctor promised to keep him peaceful. He's not peaceful!"

An efficient nurse rose to her feet and sped down the hall into your room. In a matter of minutes she had given you a shot and strapped a morphine monitor on your arm.

You closed your eyes. You stopped kicking your feet and rolling on the bed. I cried harder and, through my tears I told the nurse, "Thank you."

I put my hand on your forehead. I kissed you thinking, *it's so hard to believe your mind is gone. Maybe it isn't.* "Honey can you hear me?"

No answer.

Diane said, "He's sleeping."

I had to be thankful for that.

Diane stayed all night. There was only one place for a person to have any measure of comfort, so I went home to say our prayer alone.

The next morning I hurried to dress and be on my way to the hospital. The doctor would be there. I had to see him.

The pale green corridor seemed a mile long. I walked as fast as I could with my shoes making a loud cracking sound. I thought about how you hated that noise. The doctor had to be there. I couldn't be late. I didn't like the feel of anything.

I stepped into the room and saw Diane, hair down and rumpled, eyes tired and sad. She said, "He's been sleeping."

An aide came and spoke in a loud voice. "I need to fix his bed. And I'll see if he'll eat something."

"He's peaceful," I said. "Can't you leave him alone?"

"I won't push it too much."

Then she told me. "When you speak to him, speak loudly. He may hear you even though he can't respond."

Diane was better at that than I was. I put my face on your cheek and crying, I'd whisper, "I'm here. Honey, I'm here." Then, after a while of sobbing, I'd say to Diane, "I can't believe he doesn't know me."

Your breakfast tray sat on the table untouched. Cream of wheat, pudding and, orange juice. You wouldn't eat. You wouldn't try. Your lips cracked. Diane touched them with moistened cotton. She talked to you. She was convinced you heard.

As if sent from heaven twins came with their mother. The girls were seniors in high school.

They sang like angels, their voices filled the room and drifted down the hall. "Amazing grace how sweet the sound." Their mother put a blue Rosary against your hand and you folded your fingers around it.

The doctor came. He sat in a chair with your records, pencil and notebook. He said, "Something is taking him. I don't know what it is." He said, "It could be spinal meningitis." He wanted to know if I would give permission for a spinal tap.

I said, "No."

"Without it we will never know what took over his body."

I would allow nothing that would make you more uncomfortable.

"Medicare will not let him stay if you don't permit more treatment, more testing."

I turned to you. "We're going home." Reason told me you knew none of it, but my heart kept pounding, *I love you. I'm here.*

We contacted home-health to help with your bathing and monitoring of medication. We ordered a hospital bed. The doctor said, "Whatever is taking him is his best friend." We followed the ambulance home with the doctor's words ringing in my ears.

I'd had a large master bedroom built to take care of this eventuality--this piece of life I was forced to live. We were going home. You would sleep at the foot of our bed where we had slept together.

Diane stayed with me. We had begun the count down of your days on earth. How many would there be? How many times could I walk through the house and see you lying peacefully in our room? How many times could I touch you? How many times could I say I love you?

For three days I watched you sleeping. I put my hand on your forehead, your cheek, your lips. Through tears, I spoke to you. It was the third evening after you came home that Missy went to your bed, stood on her hind legs and peered at you through the rail. She ran around to the other side, stood up again, looked, sniffed, then hurried to her box.

It was three o'clock in the morning when I suddenly wakened. I rushed to your side. I felt your cheek. You were warm, but not breathing. Your journey had finished. Through the shadows I knew this was goodbye.

"Diane," I said, "Daddy has left us."

Jean Darby

We didn't do everything perfectly--
but we did the best we could.

About the Author

Jean Darby is the author of fifty-seven books for children, three biographies for young adults, articles, a newspaper column, and an adult novel: *Journey Out of Darkness.*

For more than two decades, her stories have excited readers in the United States and abroad—some being republished by European publishers.

Jean Darby taught school and now lectures on the skills of writing at conferences and in college classes.

She lost her husband to Alzheimer's two years ago, and from her aching but courageous heart, she wrote *I Still Love You.* It's a heartwarming story where Jean tells her husband how their days were spent during his illness.

In Jean's own invincible style she says, "My strength came quietly—as if on slippered feet."

I Still Love You is an inspiring story of love and courage.

Dr. Darby lives in Redding California. She has one daughter and four grandsons who she will gladly brag about.

Jean welcomes messages from her fans: "If you have read, *I Still Love You*, or *Journey Out of Darkness* write jeandarby@juno.com."